William May

Essay on pulmonary consumptions:

Including the histories of several remarkable instances of recovery, from the most alarming stages of the disorder, by an improved method of treatment

William May

Essay on pulmonary consumptions:
Including the histories of several remarkable instances of recovery, from the most alarming stages of the disorder, by an improved method of treatment

ISBN/EAN: 9783337714932

Printed in Europe, USA, Canada, Australia, Japan

Cover: Foto ©ninafisch / pixelio.de

More available books at **www.hansebooks.com**

ESSAY

ON

PULMONARY CONSUMPTIONS,

INCLUDING

THE HISTORIES OF

SEVERAL

REMARKABLE INSTANCES OF RECOVERY,

FROM THE MOST

ALARMING STAGES OF THE DISORDER,

BY AN

IMPROVED METHOD OF TREATMENT:

BY

WILLIAM MAY, M. D.

MEMBER OF THE ROYAL COLLEGE OF PHYSICIANS, LONDON; FELLOW OF THE LONDON MEDICAL SOCIETY; LATE ONE OF THE PHYSICIANS TO THE UNIVERSAL DISPENSARY, LONDON.

Tentanda via eft.   VIRGIL.

PLYMOUTH:

PRINTED AND SOLD BY B. HAYDON; SOLD ALSO BY CADELL, LAW, EVANS, FAULDER, LOWNDES, AND DEIGHTON, LONDON.

TO

J. COAKLEY LETTSOM, *M. D.*
F. R. S. S. A. &c. &c.

MY DEAR SIR,

IT is not merely to folicit your patronage of this work that I have infcribed it with your name, nor is it alone for the purpofe of declaring my great refpect for your character, that I have availed myfelf of this public manner of addreffing you. Defirable as your patronage certainly is, and folicitous,

upon

DEDICATION.

upon every occasion, as I am to testify my respect for the merits of your character in the public walks of science, and for the virtues which adorn it, in the sequestered vale of private life, I have yet another motive for dedicating this work to you.

As you have for many years been in possession of a most extensive practice, in the largest and most populous city in these kingdoms, and connected as you have been with many of the public charities of the metropolis, you must have had frequent and melancholy experience of the fatality of the disease which is the subject of the following dissertation

DEDICATION.

fertation. If the obfervations contained in it fhould poffefs fufficient merit to attract your attention, your extenfive expérience, and influence, will tend more fpeedily, and effectually to diffufe the good which they are calculated to produce, by fubftituting a mode of treatment that has been found eminently ufeful in many cafes, in the place of that which has feldom, if ever been found fuccefsful in a true cafe of pulmonary confumption. How it happens that it fhould have been left for thefe later days to difcover that the phthifis pulmonalis, whofe caufes and hiftory have fuffered a laborious inveftigation many centuries ago, and have occafionally employed

DEDICATION.

employed the pens of many able writers, requires a method of treatment different from that which has received the sanction of univerfal cuftom, you, who are better acquainted with the hiftory of medicine than I am, will, probably, be able to explain. It is to the dominion of prejudice that I conceive this to have been principally owing. A prejudice defcending by an hereditary fucceffion, from generation to generation, and much more ftrongly marked than the hereditary taints of gout or of fcrophula. It feems to be the genius of the prefent day to endeavor to do away fuch errors, and not to fuffer a timid apprehenfion of the poffible evils

evils of innovation, to ſtand in the way of neceſſary reform. There is certainly a preſumption in favor of any cuſtom, which through a ſucceſſion of ages, has received the ſanction of mankind. It is ſometimes, however, diſcovered that ſuch cuſtoms, though confirmed by ages, and countenanced by the authority of very wiſe, and good men, are neither generally uſeful, nor indeed founded upon principles of reaſon and juſtice. Preſuming this to have been the caſe with reſpect to the ſubject of this work, I have ventured to join my feeble efforts with thoſe which have been already made, to ſtem the torrent of this deſtructive prejudice. If they ſucceed,

ceed, in any degree, with the public, I shall be highly gratified, and if they prove satisfactory to you, I shall still enjoy the higher pleasure arising from the praise that is worth ambition, "*laudari a laudatis viris.*"

Among the many public instances of your liberality, the zealous support you have given to the numerous public charities which do the highest honor to the benevolent spirit of this nation, is very conspicuous. The Alderfgate, Public, and Finfbury Dispensaries are greatly indebted to your exertions; the Humane Society will long remain a memorial of your indefatigable zeal

in

DEDICATION.

in the caufe of humanity, and public happinefs; and the London Medical Society has found in you a moft liberal patron, and an active and ufeful member. While I feel much obligation to you, in common with the members of our profeffion, and fociety in general, on thefe accounts, I am alfo peculiarly indebted to you for many inftances of private friendfhip with which you have honored me. Retired, as I now am, from the wide field of London practice, to a circle better fuited to the exercife of my humble talents, though I am debarred from the pleafure and advantage of immediate intercourfe with you, I fhall ftill hope for the continuance of

your

DEDICATION.

your friendship, which I will constantly endeavor to cultivate, and which it will be my pride and happiness to preserve as long as I live.

I am, dear sir, with great esteem,

your obliged and faithful friend

and obedient servant,

WILLIAM MAY.

PLYMOUTH,
BROAD-STREET,
March 1, 1792.

INTRODUCTION.

A perfuafion of the incurable nature of Confumptions of the Lungs, which has fo generally prevailed amongft perfons of all defcriptions, appears to have thrown very confiderable obftacles in the way of improving the treatment of this cruel difeafe. In the firft inftance, the medical world acting under the influence of this perfuafion, the induftry of enquiry has been checked, and very little progrefs has been made in the attempts to afcertain either the true nature of the difeafe, or the moft rational,

rational, and effectual methods of curing it. That ardor of investigation, which, upon other occasions, has excited the exertions of the most industrious, and ingenious medical writers of the present age, seems to have been damped by the chilling conviction of the unavoidable fatality of a disease, of which the best knowledge to be obtained, was but imperfect, and in the treatment of which, the best appropriated medicines had been hitherto unsuccessful. This sentiment, baneful in its operation, and I hope erroneous in its foundation, has been held,

with

with few exceptions, by medical men for a feries of years: on the other hand, people in general, biaffed by the opinion of thofe who alone can be competent judges of the important queftion, and obferving, as it too frequently happens, the fatal event of the complaint, even where the earlieft, and the moft efficacious methods of cure had apparently been adopted, imbibe the fame perfuafion. The confequence of this, for the moft part, is the neglect of that fpeedy application for relief, which affords the moft reafonable expectation of fuccefs;

success; and a despondency succeeds which spreads its contagious influence generally amongst all the friends of the patient, who is considered by them as a victim devoted to certain, and inevitable destruction.

It seems, however, to have been wisely, and humanely ordered by Divine Providence, that the patient himself should be kept out of the reach of the pernicious contagion of this sentiment of despondency and terror: he either feels in reality the certain hope of recovery, or, desirous of giving solace to those

whose

whofe anxiety diftreffes him, affumes the fallacious appearance of that hope, while probably, the opinion which they have inculcated, and which the almoft univerfal prejudice of mankind has confirmed, of the impoffibility of recovery, is preying upon his mind, at once fhortening, and embittering the refidue of his life. To combat this deftructive prejudice, and to endeavor to eftablifh an opinion, which I profefs to entertain, that there exifts a method of curing the pulmonary confumption, even in its moft advanced ftage, is the intention

tion with which I am about to pub-
lifh this effay: and let me not
haftily be accufed with having ar-
rogantly, and prefumptuoufly under-
taken it; for the authorities on
my fide, though not numerous,
are ftrong, and fuch as carry, in my
mind, conviction along with them.
Independently of fpeculative and
theoretical doctrines on the fubject,
the facts which I have in my pof-
feffion will, I hope, afford confirmation ftrong of the propriety of my
opinion; and as thefe facts are not
adduced from my own obfervation
only, but collected from the writings

ings and communications of thofe whofe ability to afcertain the precife nature of the difeafe, is unqueftionable, and whofe veracity, and integrity of intention, are totally unimpeachable, whoever refufes to give them entire credit, will hardly avoid the imputation of an obftinate, dangerous, and criminal fcepticifm of character.

It has been well obferved by an intelligent and elegant writer,* that to pronounce a difeafe incurable, is frequently to make it fo; nor can the

* Vide Gregory's "Duties and Offices of a Phyfician."

the opinion that there is no difeafe in its nature abfolutely irremediable, bring the charge of arrogance upon any one who profeffes to maintain it, if he is modeft enough, at the fame time, to admit that there may exift difeafes which he does not know how to cure. This is the acceptation in which I would wifh to underftand the term incurable. I am not willing to admit that it implies, in any cafe, a pofitive irremediable quality in the difeafe, but would apply it only to exprefs our imperfect knowledge, and erroneous practice in the treatment of thofe difeafes, for which no remedy has hitherto been difcovered. That the phthifis pulmonalis is not to be reckoned among this number, I truſt I ſhall be able abundantly to convince any candid and liberal reader. Thofe of a different defcription, into whofe hands this work may chance to fall, to whofe praife or cenfure I am equally indifferent, may confider the pofition which I wifh to eftablifh, as fpeculative and vifionary, and doubt the authenticity of the facts upon which it is founded. They may alfo, perhaps, go a ſtep farther, and confider my belief of the doctrine I am defirous of inculcating, to arife from a credulity which is the concomitant of ignorance. A vice, which however frequent in common life, is, I think, lefs frequently to be obferved in the medical department, than in any other. *"Damnant quod non intelligunt,"* is much more applicable to the uninformed part of medical practitioners, than the charge of a ready belief of it. If I fhould happen to incur this imputation of credulity, to ufe the fentiment, and language of a very learned and fenfible writer, it will fit very eafy upon me, as it is, for the

the moſt part, found to proceed from men who have no other meaſure of probability than their own very limited experience, or ſome lame and defective theory, eſpouſed without any experience at all.

To thoſe, for inſtance, who believe that an ulcer of the lungs is univerſally incurable, the caſes which I have to deſcribe may appear to have been fabricated, for the mere purpoſe of furniſhing a declamatory eſſay, or ſome other unworthy motive. And yet, in a great variety of caſes, it has been incontrovertibly

incontrovertibly proved, that the lungs have been fhot through by mufket bullets, or otherwife materially wounded, fo as to occafion inflammation, fuppuration, and a long train of evil confequences, from which the moft perfect recovery has been obtained. There is fcarcely a furgeon in the army or navy, of any confiderable experience in his profeffion, to whom fuch cafes have not occurred. One inftance of this kind, which has never yet been publifhed, affords a proof irrefragable of the fact, and is of fo interefting a nature, and fo very appofite polite to my present purpose, that I shall subjoin it in a note, without any further apology.*

Without

* A gentleman, during the American war, was under the unfortunate necessity of meeting a brother officer in a duel. The shot of his antagonist entered his breast, passing in the direction of the right lobe of the lungs, thro' which it appeared to have penetrated. The external hæmorrhage was not very considerable, but a large quantity of blood was expectorated, accompanied with great difficulty of breathing; and a cough, and symptoms of violent inflammation, speedily supervened. The antiphlogistic regimen was adopted, and every judicious method of obviating inflammatory diathesis was assiduously used. Blood continued to be discharged, by coughing, for many days, which was followed by a truly purulent expectoration, and all the symptoms of a perfect pulmonary consumption. The exact duration of these complaints I cannot now ascertain;

symptoms

Without any violent breach of

symptoms of convalescence, however, soon appeared, and the patient entirely recovered from the injury he had received. During the purulent expectoration, a circumstance occurred, which places the actual injury which the lungs themselves had sustained, beyond all possibility of doubt. A piece of flannel cloth was thrown up by the cough, enveloped in a clot of blood and pus, and upon comparing it with a hole in an inner waistcoat, through which the bullet had passed, it was found exactly to correspond with it, and had been actually carried along with the ball into the cavity of the wounded lung: The ball continued its progress, and passing out between the ribs of the posterior part of the chest, was afterwards extracted from the region of the loins, where it had descended by its own gravity, and deposited itself just beneath the common integuments.*

* I am indebted to my friend Mr. Adams, of Liskeard, an ingenious Surgeon of the Navy, for this communication, who was himself an eye witness of this seemingly extraordinary circumstance.

nofological privilege, the cafe related below might be denominated a perfect pulmonary confumption. I have the authority of Sauvage, who has claffed the phthifis ab vulnere amongft the varieties of this difeafe which he has enumerated. And furely it muft be admitted, that this was a cafe of a pretty formidable kind, clearly and decidedly poffeffing every fymptom, independently of a peculiar diathefis of the fyftem, hereafter to be confidered, which can be neceffary to characterize a true and exquifite phthifis pulmonalis. All the danger that

that can be fuppofed to arife from impeded circulation, ruptured blood veffels, extenfive inflammation of a vital organ, from its fuppuration, and all that could be apprehended from the confinement, and abforption of the pus which was generated, was prefent in the cafe already cited. And to thofe who eftimate the danger, in fuch cafes, to be in proportion to the tendency in the conftitution to an inflammatory difpofition, this patient will appear to have labored under the further difadvantages of a robuft and firm habit: notwithftanding all which difadvantages,

advantages, affording perhaps as gloomy a prognoſtic as can well be imagined, the diſeaſe was happily removed, and the patient reſtored to as good a ſtate of health as he had ever previouſly enjoyed.

It would ſwell to too great a bulk this part of the work, which I find already to exceed the limits with which I intended to circumſcribe it, were I to enumerate all the caſes in my recollection, which bear a ſtriking reſemblance to that above mentioned. Many of them are already to be found in the records of the profeffion, and of others I fhall occafionally make mention in the progrefs of this effay. Before, however, I quit this part of the fubject, I muft recur for a moment, to the hiftory of the cafe which I have related, as an illuftration of a very important fact, with refpect to the nature, treatment, and event of confumptions in general, appears to me very clearly to arife from it.

In the patient whofe hiftory I have given, no evidence appears of any morbid tendency affecting the fyftem, (except the exiftence of firm, elaftic, elaſtic, and robuſt muſcular fibres can be ſuppoſed to conſtitute ſuch a morbid diſpoſition*) either preceding, or accompanying the diſeaſe.

It is a contaminated habit of body, ſome latent vitiated principle in the conſtitution, upon which the fatality of conſumptions has depended; and whatever tends to correct

---

* Some recent doctrines, founded, I am afraid, more in hypotheſis, than truth, have taught that a "high degree of good health, is, in fact, no more than a prediſpoſition to diſeaſe." *Proclivitas ad diatheſin ſthenicam*; and this curious ſoleciſm has been very warmly, and very ably ſupported by its advocates.

rect that principle, and to improve the general habit of the conſtitution, will be found beſt appropriated to the cure of phthiſis. I maintain that it is upon this principle alone the diſeaſe is ever likely to be remedied, and that the vulnerary, balſamic, and expectorating medicines, which have been given with a view of ſpecifically operating upon the affected organs, have been vainly, and fooliſhly adminiſtered. I do not mean to contend that the claſſes of vulnerary, balſamic, and expectorating medicines, are under all circumſtances, of no utility, though

though I confefs my doubts of the general efficacy which has been afcribed to them. It is to this application only, with the view to produce thefe fpecific effects upon ulcerations of the lungs, that I object. This practice was firft adopted when the knowledge of the animal œconomy was exceedingly limited and imperfect. I take it for granted, that there are very few practitioners of the prefent day, who will believe that Peruvian Balfam, (or any other balfamic, or vulnerary medicine,) adminiftered for the cure of an ulcer of the lungs, can

can be conveyed to the affected part, and act there, in its original and proper form, quafi Peruvian Balfam. In the ftomach it has a very formidable progrefs to undergo, by which, moft probably, it is totally deprived of its original form and quality, before it is at all diftributed to the other parts of the body. And when this diftribution does take place, it is not poffible that any partial determination of it can happen, fo as to affect the lungs rather than any other part of the body: for having entered, thro' its proper channels, into the blood veffels, vessels, it is equally, and impartially diffused, throughout the whole system; and the remotest parts are equally subject to its operation, with those that are more contiguous; for the contiguity of the lungs with the stomach, hath nothing at all to do with the operation of these, or, indeed, of any other remedies. The medium of communication is not affected by the contiguity of parts, but extends itself to all the organized parts of the body; it is in fact commensurate with the extent of the nervous and vascular systems, and affords as ready

ready a communication with the remoteſt extremities of the body, as it does with the centre.

I ſhall apologize for this digreſ-ſion, by inſerting a quotation from the work of a very ingenious writer, which applies very forcibly to the ſubject under our conſideration. "Remarkable inſtances of the ſpontaneous cure of very conſiderable injuries of the lungs are ſometimes ſeen, not only where the injury is received in a ſtate of health, with a good habit of body, and where there is an active diſpoſition in the conſtitution conftitution to remedy accidental defects, but we are not without examples where confiderable complaints of the lungs, which had taken their rife from, or at leaft during a fault of the conftitution, have, however, upon a falutary alteration in the habit, healed of themfelves."*

The abfence of this morbid taint of the conftitution, and, in my opinion, that alone, furnifhes the diftinction between cafes of accidental injury,

* Vide Mudge's Radical Cure for a Catarrhous Cough. P. 75.

injury, similar to that which has been recited, and those alarming diseases of the lungs, the very name of which carries terror and consumption along with it; the treatment of which, founded as I trust I shall be able to prove, upon a lame and defective theory of the disease, and co-operating with that destructive persuasion of its unavoidable fatality, which is equally to be lamented, and deprecated, has materially contributed to the opprobrium which the science of medicine and its professors have suffered upon the occasion, through a succession ceffion of ages; from the time of Hippocrates, to that of the great Boerhaave, and down to the ftill more enlightened days of Huxham and Cullen.

Juftly celebrated as thefe great characters have been for their great genius, extenfive experience, and indefatigable induftry, in the improvement of the fcience of medicine, I may reafonably expect to be accufed of arrogance, and prefumption, in attempting to effect that which the united efforts of fuch wonderful abilities have failed to perform.

perform. It is not without some terrors of this kind that I have been prompted to make such an attempt: while, however, I have the sanction of such an authority as Dr. Percival, for the ground work of the undertaking, whose philosophical and intelligent mind, joined with uncommon professional knowledge, and endowed with the best habits of observation, and whose zeal for promoting the interest and happiness of society, has never been exceeded, I am sure that the design, at least, cannot want any apology. I have also the satisfaction to observe

Doctor

Doctor Kentifh, and many other very refpectable labourers, in the fame field; and if my endeavor tofurnifh any ufeful information on the fubject, to practitioners, fhould be found ineffectual, it may probably produce the effect of exciting others, of more competent ability, to undertake it; and as the advancement of profeffional knowledge, and the benefit which muft neceffarily accrue to fociety, from whatever tends to improve the practice of medicine, are the principal objects which I have in view, in either cafe, the end of this publication

lication will be answered, and I shall be amply gratified.

As it is not my design to write a systematic treatise on the subject of pulmonary consumption, I would wish to anticipate any objections which may be made to the desultory nature of this essay, by informing my readers, that I mean to confine myself principally to the consideration of the nosological character of the disease, and to practical observations founded upon that basis. Those who are desirous of going farther into the subject, will find

find some very ingenious speculations in the writings of Dr. Reid, and a very elaborate and accurate history of the disease in Dr. Cullen's First Lines of the Practice of Physic; and for further information, with respect to the causes, and treatment of the disease, I would recommend them to consult an admirable work on Phthisis, lately published by Dr. Michael Ryan, and the ingenious essay of my learned friend Dr. Simmons, entitled " Practical Observations on Consumptions." The writings, also, of the late excellent Dr. Musgrave contain some useful hints

hints respecting this disease, of which I should have taken particular notice, if I had been so fortunate as to meet with them* before this work went to the press. As, however, I mean to pursue the consideration of this subject, in a future work, I shall certainly avail myself of some of the observations of this great man, whose premature death was an irreparable loss to society, and has been severely felt, and sincerely lamented, by the medical science in particular, as well as the whole republic of literary men.

* Gulstonian Lectures, &c. by Samuel Musgrave, M.D. F. R. S. &c. Physician at Plymouth.

CHAP. 1.

I shall first proceed to enumerate a few cases, in order to confirm the fact which I am desirous of establishing, both with respect to the possibility, and method of cure, of consumptive cases. Some of these have come under my own immediate observation; some are extracted from publications on the subject, the characters of the authors of which, will be a sufficient testimony of their authenticity; for others I am indebted to several gentlemen of the profession, who have had the goodness to communicate to me the result of their experience. In this part of my work I have been solicitous to observe brevity, rather than to exercise the patience of my readers, by a prolix detail of all the cases which I might have related; as I take it for granted, that a few well attested facts, will afford as ample a testimony of the point which they are calculated to ascertain, as a thousand.

I have been solicitous, also, rather to avail myself of the authorities of others, than to insist upon my own experience, in the support of my doctrine. Those cases which have been related in their naked simplicity, without any suspicion of the use that might be made of them, cannot reasonably be charged with unfairness, or partiality, and while they are unimpeachable in this respect, the reputation of the authors of them will

effectually

effectually fecure them againſt any fufpicion that their true nature has been in any degree mifunderſtood, or mifreprefented.

In an ingenious eſſay on the utility of fwinging in the treatment of confumptions, by Dr Carmichael Smyth, many inſtances are related of cafes fuccefsfully treated, in which, from the duration and formidable fymptoms of the difeafe, the death of the patient feemed unavoidable. In other publications of a recent date, inſtances are alfo to be found of the happy event of fuch cafes as precluded the reafonable expectation of recovery. The inaugural diſſertation of my friend and colleague Dr Kentiſh,* exhibits

---

* Vide Diſſ. Inaugural: de Phthifi Pulmonali Auctore R. Kentiſh. Edinburgh, edit: Anno 1784. When the avocations

hibits a wonderful inftance of the recovery of a gentleman, who was a ftudent of medicine at Edinburgh, under the moft alarming fymptoms of a phthifis pulmonalis, attended with emaciation, purulent fpitting, and hectic fever. The Memoirs of the London Medical Society* contain fome remarks by Dr Tho. Percival of Manchefter, peculiarly applicable to the general fcope of this publication. — Two cafes are related of pulmonary confumptions ending favourably, under a mode of treatment which I fhall take notice of in another place. One of them is defcribed, from Dr. Percival's own obfervation of Dr. Kentifh fhall allow him leifure to profecute the fubject which he is fo exceedingly well qualified to elucidate and improve, the public may expect another, and a more elaborate work, on the interefting fubject of the prefent enquiry.

* Vide Medical Cautions and Remarks. Memoirs of the Medical Society of London, V. II.

obfervation, to have been, in the common acceptation of the language, a gallopping confumption.

Dr. Mudge of Plymouth, in his philofophical, and excellent differtation on the Catarrhous Cough, has given the hiftory of an extraordinary cafe of phthifis, which occured at St. Thomas's Hofpital; an account of which I fhall fubjoin, in another part of this work, in the words of the author. To thefe I muft add the hiftory of an alarming difeafe of the fame kind, which fell under my own obfervation, an account of which, with fome nofological remarks not neceffary to be repeated here, has already been publifhed in the London Medical Journal for the year 1788.—I fhall recite the cafe with as much

much brevity as it will admit of. The patient was a girl about eighteen years old; had a narrow cheſt, high ſhoulders, a long neck, fine ſkin, with a peculiar whiteneſs and tranſparency of the teeth; together with a circumſcribed redneſs of the cheeks, and other appearances indicating, in general, a predifpofition to phthifis, and was born of fcrophulous parents.

About eight or ten weeks before I ſaw her, ſhe was firſt feized with a cough, which was apparently of a catarrhous kind; It was extremely urgent, without expectoration, and accompanied, from time to time, with flight pains affecting varioufly the thorax, but confined to no particular part of it. She had alfo complained occafionally of irregular rigors,

rigors, followed by heat, and flushing of the face.

After a few weeks passed away in this manner, the symptoms, by slow degrees, growing more and more troublesome, a frothy mucus was expectorated, which was sometimes tinged with blood. In a short time, this hæmorrhage became more considerable, and recurred pretty regularly, at the stated period of four or five days. It was constantly preceded by those symptoms which are usually found to accompany the hæmorrhagic effort in similar cases: namely, a titillation of the fauces, flushing of the face, dyspnoea, and a disagreeable sense of burning in the chest, with an increased frequency, and apparent hardness of the pulse.*

These

* Vide Cullens Synopsis Nosologiæ Methodicæ. Tom. 2d. P. 196.

These symptoms were always relieved by the ceasing of the hæmorrhage, and in the intervals between the attack, the same kind of mucous matter as has been above described, continued to be expectorated. At length the sputum increased considerably in quantity, put on an evident appearance of purulency, and the symptoms of pyrexia became more strongly marked.

It was at this period of the disease when I first visited the patient. She was then in a state of extreme weakness, with her face shrunk, and the whole body exceedingly emaciated. The noon and evening exacerbations of hectic fever, with profuse sweats, recurred in a very regular succession. The bowels were sometimes constipated; at others they

they were affected with profusely colliquative discharges, which, while they lasted, lessened the discharge by the skin. The consent between the skin, and the intestinal canal, was very clearly evinced in this instance, in which these different conditions of the bowels alternated with each other, with great regularity. The pulse, in point of frequency, was irregular, but invariably above a hundred and ten; sometimes, especially before the hæmorrhage, somewhat full and hard, but for the most part, small, and extremely weak. The matter expectorated was now considerable in quantity, and by the common criteria, as well as those of Dr. Brugmans,* and the late Mr. Charles Darwin, appeared very

---

* Vide Dissertatio Inauguralis de Puogenia. Auct. D. Brugmans, M. D. Botanices Leidæ Professore.

very satisfactorily, to be of a purulent nature. Her nights were anxious and restless, her breathing laborious and painful, and if kept out of bed but a few hours, her legs became oedematous. She had the pearly whiteness of the tunica adnata of the eye, the adunque incurvated form of the nails, and the defluxio capillorum which Sydenham, Cullen, and other writers have considered as certain diagnostics with respect to the existence of a confirmed pulmonary consumption. It will, I think, be allowed, that it is hardly possible to imagine a case more perfectly defined than the above related, or more unfavorable of its kind; a more threatening assemblage of symptoms could scarcely have combined, in any disease, to furnish a dismal prognostic of impending danger; notwithstanding which, a perfect cure was obtained, by a mode of treatment which I shall describe in the sequel, and the patient has now enjoyed, for the space of several years, a firm, and uninterrupted state of health.

In the last volume of the same work* in which this account was first printed, a case of a similar nature has been published, which, though the event was not equally fortunate, affords so striking a proof of the efficacy of the mode of treatment which I have recommended, upon the principles hereafter to be explained, and operates so powerfully in support of the doctrine contained in this essay, that I cannot pass it over in silence. A lady, aged about twenty-three, of a florid complexion,

* Vide London Medical Journal, Vol. 11th. P. 388.

complexion, and clear fkin, with a fomewhat enlarged thyroid gland, but no other diftinguifhing marks of fcrophula, had returned from Briftol, in an hopelefs ftate of apparently confirmed phthifis pulmonalis. She labored under extreme debility, languor, and emaciation; a violent, troublefome, and inceffant cough, preceded by hæmoptyfis, and attended with a copious expectoration of purulent matter: a hectic fever, with regular exacerbations, night fweats, and a great tendency to diarrhoea. She had little fleep, and experienced a total lofs of appetite and ftrength; indeed, the laft was fo far exhaufted, that fhe was under the neceffity of being carried to, and from her bed, and was utterly incapable of ftanding without fupport. Her cafe appeared (from the defcription of

the

the author,* in whofe words I am defcribing it,) fo truly deplorable and helplefs, as would have juftified any medical man, in pronouncing her diffolution to be at hand. The pulfe, though as quick as a hundred and thirty-four in a minute, yet was extremely low and weak, and the whole fyftem in a ftate of debility. A tonic plan of treatment was adopted, owing to the recollection of the remarks which I had publifhed in the London Medical Journal, on the fubject of a fimilar cafe already mentioned, which were then frefh in the author's memory. The faline draughts, and emulfions which fhe had been previoufly ufing without effect, were thrown afide, the antiphlogiftic treatment,

* Mr. Edmund Pitts Gapper, of Mere, Wiltfhire.

ment, which had hitherto been purſued, was abandoned, and draughts, compounded of a ſtrong decoction of red bark, aromatic confection, and compound tincture of lavender, were ſubſtituted. A little cinnamon, and Gum Arabic were added to the decoction, to obviate any tendency to diarrhoea. A ſufficient quantity of tincture of opium was adminiſtered, every night, to procure ſleep, and was increaſed, by degrees, without the leaſt inconvenience, to ſeventy drops at each doſe. It was alſo recommended to her, to make uſe of a more invigorating regimen than ſhe had hitherto done; ſhe was enjoined to take frequently, nay every hour, a ſmall quantity of ſome nouriſhing food, ſuch as ſago, ſalep, tapioca, jellies, chicken and mutton broths; ſhe was allowed a light

animal

animal food dinner, and to drink three or four glaſſes of wine in the courſe of the day, and even in the night, at convenient intervals: She was carried out in a ſedan chair, whenever the weather permitted, for a few minutes at each time; increaſing it by degrees, as her ſtrength allowed. This plan was perſiſted in upwards of two months, and the effects were as follow. The pulſe, in the ſpace of a week, came down to a hundred; in three weeks to ninety; and finally, to near its natural ſtandard. As the frequency of the pulſe abated, ſo did the fever, till it entirely left her. The expectoration grew gradually leſs in quantity, and at laſt conſiſted chiefly, but not entirely, of phlegm. She had comfortable nights, her appetite and ſtrength returned, and the latter in ſo eminent

nent a degree, as to enable her to walk frequently in the garden, without any affiftance, and to ride on horfeback, fingle, twice every day.*

The cafe related by Dr. Kentifh, alluded to in the former part of this chapter, I fhall fubjoin in his own words. *" Unus ex amicis meis, Raius Beckwith, quum febre hectica, tuffi violenta, exfcreatione purulenta, fudoribus colliquativis*

---

* The ultimate event of this cafe, (which Mr. Gapper has related with a degree of accuracy and candor, that does him great honor,) as being unconnected with the fubject immediately before us, is not neceffary to be mentioned here. I cannot, however, difmifs the confideration of this cafe, without obferving, that the obfervations annexed to it, are made with great fpirit and judgement, and are well entitled to the attention of practitioners.

liquativis diu laborassfet; diæta parca lactea, sine fructu, tandem, contra medici consilium, victu pleniore, ostraeis, Falerno, et cerevisia, usus est: symptomata maligna disparuerunt, feliciterque convaluebat."*

Doctor Mudge's account of a cafe, which does not materially differ from the above, is as follows. Speaking of the examples of phthifis, either produced by, or attended with, a contaminated habit of body, having been fometimes cured by fuch means as have been found to produce a falutary alteration in the conftitution, he fays, " An extraordinary cafe of this fort I remember once to have feen in St. Thomas's Hofpital, in a patient

---

* Vide Differt. De Phthifi Pulmonali Auct. R. Kentifh; Edinburgh, 1784.

patient of Sir Edward Wilmott's. Whether the diforder began before his admiffion, or commenced during his refidence in the hofpital, I do not now recollect, but the man, however, fell into a pulmonary phthifis. After fpitting off large quantities of pus, attended with a hectic fever, and colliquative fweats, he was at laft reduced to fo weak and emaciated a ftate, that all probability of phyfical relief being at an end, and his death daily expected, he ceafed being particularly attended to, at the ordinary vifits of the ward. The man, however, lived on; and at laft, contrary to the expectation of every one, the difeafe feemed not only not to gain ground, but appeared to afford fome flight indications of a poffibility of recovery. The purulent difcharge evidently abated; his night fweats sweats were less profuse; the quick and palpitating pulse began to be more quiet and distinct; and some little appetite returning, his countenance and eyes seemed to promise some hopes of returning life. These very extraordinary and unexpected appearances engaged the attention of his physician, who recommended a diet suited to his circumstances, and advised him to remove into the country. About three quarters of a year after, this very patient was again admitted into the hospital, for a complaint in his leg, though otherwise in perfect health; and during his residence there, was unfortunately seized with the small-pox, and died. As his former cure had been so very singular, the body was opened, when it appeared, that during his consumptive complaints, the

greatest

greateſt part of the right lobe of the lungs had been totally deſtroyed, and that, conſequently, reſpiration had been principally performed by the left."*

In

---

* Vide a Radical Cure, &c. by J. Mudge, F. R. S. &c. Plymouth, p. 76. In a communication with which Doctor Mudge has favored me on this ſubject, which I feel it to be my duty, in point of candor, to annex to the above quotation, he ſtates his opinion " that this caſe aſcertains, or was intended to prove, nothing, but that the renovating powers of Nature were ſufficient to eſtabliſh health, when the original cauſe of the diſeaſe had ceaſed to exiſt." What the caſe, as it is related in this very excellent diſſertation, was intended to prove, is certainly of no conſequence to the purpoſe of this publication; but with reſpect to the fact contained in it, I humbly conceive, that it aſcertains two points of very material conſequence to the diſeaſe under our conſideration; firſt, that in a moſt advanced, and dangerous

ſtage,

In Morton's Phthifiologia, a work publifhed in the former part of this century, there

ftage, it is not incurable ; and, fecondly, upon the fuppofition that the treatment adopted in the firft inftance, was of the antiphlogiftic complexion of thofe days, (of which, indeed, though I have not obtained any pofitive evidence, there is a very ftrong prefumption,) it afcertains, that the remiffion of this treatment, and the neceffary fuccedaneum of common nourifhment, accompanied with change of air, and exercife, proved a fuccefsful method of cure. With refpect, alfo, to the mode in which the cure was effected, I muft take the liberty to differ, in fome meafure, from the ingenious author of the above-mentioned work ; or, at leaft, to fuggeft a conftruction fomewhat different from that which he appears to have given it. The doctrine of proximate caufes teaches us, that the proximate caufe of any difeafe, conftitutes in fact, the difeafe itfelf. For example, in pneumonia, an increafed tone, and action of the veffels of the lungs, or pleura, attended with an inflammatory diathefis

of

there are several instances recorded of the succefsful treatment of consumptions, by tonic

of the syftem, is the proximate caufe of the difeafe. Again, in phthifis, a peculiar contamination of the habit, accompanied with, or producing tubercles, or ulceration of the lungs, is the proximate caufe of the difeafe. In either cafe, the ceafing of the original caufe is the cure of the difeafe; and it is to the removal of this caufe that all the endeavors of medicine are directed. When this is effected, the powers of Nature muft neceffarily re-eftablifh health, the obftacles in the way of thefe renovating powers being removed, as foon as ever the proximate caufe of any difeafe has ceafed to exift. If I have been fo fortunate as to exprefs my meaning with perfpicuity on this fubject, it will convey an opinion which I wifh to be clearly intelligible; namely, that to remove the impediments to the falutary operation of Nature, is a very important part of the indication of cure in all difeafes. This doctrine has been inculcated by an authority as great as Hippocrates himfelf, and the increafing experience of every day confirms

tonic means; but the abfurd theories with which the facts are encumbered, are fo numerous and tedious, that it would be as irkfome, as it is unneceffary to relate them.

The following cafe has been communicated to me by a Surgeon of Eaft Looe, of great ability and veracity.

A

confirms its propriety. The Vis Medicatrix Naturæ is a moft powerful agent in the cure of difeafes: To obviate the difficulties in the way of its exertions, is the moft rational part of the fcience of medicine, and when this is accomplifhed, with fuch effectual affiftances, as we are enabled to adminifter to its operations, I hope I am not too fanguine in expecting, that even in the moft hopelefs cafes, as it happened in that above related, we fhall have it in our power to apply to this falutary agent, what has been faid of Truth *Magna eft et prævalebit.*

A young woman living in the parifh of Pelynt, of a phthifical habit of body, was affected with a cough, purulent fpitting, profufe fweats, and hectic fever, attended with great emaciation of the body. Thefe complaints had been of confiderable duration, and were preceded, in the firft inftance, by the common fymptoms of an incipient ftage of pulmonary confumption. Before, however, any medical affiftance was afforded her, the diforder was arrived at an advanced ftage, and night fweats had fo exhaufted the patient, that her recovery feemed to be altogether an impoffible event. With the idea, therefore, of palliating only thofe evils, the removal of which appeared to be beyond the powers of medicine, an opiate was adminiftered, (*illud divinum*, as Dr. Huxham has exprefled preſſed it, *miſcrorum ſolamen,*) towards evening, and occaſionally during the day, to alleviate the cough, which harraſſed and wore out the patient. Theſe palliatives had the deſired effect, and afforded an opportunity of adminiſtering other medicines with the hope of advantage. Bliſters were applied to the ſides, and other parts of the cheſt, to relieve the pain, and difficulty of breathing; myrrh was alſo given, with the ſquill pill, and a mixture compoſed of the volatile alkali, and oil, in the form of an emulſion, to promote expectoration; the bark at the ſame time was liberally uſed; with theſe medicines, the means of ſupporting and nouriſhing the body were made uſe of, and under this mode of treatment, the patient, in the ſpace of two months, reco-

veſed

vered perfectly from her difeafe, and is now a very healthy woman, and the mother of feveral children.

To thofe which have been mentioned, I fhall add two other cafes which have occurred to me, fince my firft publication on the fubject, of which the fymptoms were equally well marked, and the event alike fortunate. The firft was a patient under the care of

Note. Mr. Coytmor, an ingenious Surgeon of Eaft Looe, has informed me, that he has been in the habit of ufing a tonic method of treatment, in confumptive cafes, for many years, and has meet with feveral inftances of its good effects. One Jago, of the parifh of Pelint, had labored under the fymptoms of a pulmonary phthifis, for fome time, and was effectually cured by a nourifhing regimen, the ufe of fome ftomachic bitters, and pills, compofed of fquills, ginger, ammoniacum, and very fmall dofes of calomel.

of Mr. Pearce, a judicious apothecary of St. Kevern, in Cornwall. A man, aged about thirty, of a thin and weakly habit of body, had been affected, for feveral weeks, with cough, difficulty of breathing, and expectoration of offenfive matter, accompanied with great wafting of the body, night fweats, and a confirmed hectic fever. Previous to the attack of thefe fymptoms, his health had been, for the fpace of feveral months, very much impaired. His appetite was gone; his bowels were occafionally affected with a feemingly colliquative purging, but generally coftive. His countenance was pale and emaciated, his eyes funk, with the tunica conjunctiva of a colour characteriftic of his hectic condition, and the whole body exhibited the appearance of extreme weaknefs

nefs, which the debility and frequency of his pulfe confirmed. An emetic of ipecacuanha was given, and repeated at intervals, while the bark and myrrh, both in fubftance and infufion, were daily adminiftered. A mild opiate was exhibited at nights, to relieve his dyfpnoea, and to obviate other fpafmodic conftrictions of the thorax, as well as to allay the irritation of coughing. A blifter, alfo, was applied to the cheft, with good effect. The bowels were treated as the circumftances of conftipation or relaxation required, and fuch light and nutritious food was allowed him, as fuited the weak condition of the organs of digeftion; wine was alfo taken in moderate quantities, to obviate the languor, and excite the energy of the fyftem. This plan, perfevered in for the

fpace

ON PULMONARY CONSUMPTIONS. 29

space of five or six weeks, with variations accommodated to little changes in his complaint, quite unneceffary to be taken notice of here, effectually removed the difeafe: and though I am not willing to conceal that, during the latter part of his treatment, he took fome dofes of a famous cordial, fold, and faid to be invented, by one Godbold, a notorious vender of medicine in London, I cannot be perfuaded that the medicines above defcribed, the falutary effects of which I had an opportunity of noticing, were not wholly entitled to the credit of his cure.

The other cafe was a young man, of the name of Fowle, whom I attended, in confultation with Mr. Pout, Surgeon, of Yalding, in Kent. He had been ill about two months,

months, with the common symptoms of an incipient phthisis pulmonalis, which seemed to have been produced originally by exposure to cold and moisture, during a fatiguing journey. He was of a delicate constitution, and possessed, very evidently, a scrophulous habit of body. Various medicines, consisting principally of the demulcent, and expectorant class, had been tried previous to my visiting him, but with no lasting good effect. His cough was distressing; oppression of the chest was a very troublesome symptom, and this was attended with erratic pains in the side, for which, but for the contra-indication of his scrophulous habit, and the great debility indicated by the frequency and weakness of the pulse, I should have thought a small bleeding very adviseable.

On

On thefe accounts, and from a conviction that the oppreffion and pain which he fuffered, could have been produced, under fuch circumftances, by a fpafmodic affection only, I preferred the application of a blifter, and flannel waiftcoat. I ordered him to ride on horfeback every day, or as often, and as far as his ftrength would permit him. I recommended, at the fame time, a tonic, and antifpafmodic draught, compofed of the decoction, and tincture of bark, with tincture of lavender, and caftor, to be ufed twice or thrice a day, and an anodyne draught, with a fmall portion of antimonial wine, to be taken at bed-time. He was alfo directed to make ufe of a light animal food regimen, from which he had been debarred by the miftaken kindnefs of his friends, and to drink occafionally occasionally a small draught of wine or porter. The state of his bowels was attended to, in the mean time, and kept soluble by means of rhubarb, and tincture of senna. A speedy alteration for the better took place, and persisting in the application of the remedies prescribed, in the space of a very few weeks he thoroughly recovered.

Having now dwelt, with too great prolixity, I fear, upon the recital of those cases which I have conceived necessary to establish the curable nature of many very formidable diseases, to which the appellation of consumption is with great justice applied, I shall proceed to enquire into the connexion which this disease has with a scrophulous habit of body, which will lead to the consideration of of the mode of treatment generally adopted, and to the elucidation of the principles upon which, in the inſtances related, I have ventured to differ from the eſtabliſhed practice.

CHAP. 2d.

HOW ſcrophula was firſt produced, or to what cauſes its propagation has been owing, is not ſo much the ſubject of the preſent enquiry, as it is to aſcertain its extenſive influence, and to mark the ſymptoms by which it is diſtinguiſhed. If in the progreſs of this enquiry, the analogy between ſcrophula

scrophula and consumption of the lungs should appear to be evident, or if a strong presumption only should arise, that a predisposition to the latter disease is materially connected with a scrophulous diathesis of the system, I conceive that great light will thereby be thrown upon the treatment of it, which I have presumed to recommend, and that the principles upon which it is founded will bear the test of severest scrutiny. If it should further appear that the diseases are uniformly and invariably connected, that they have originated in the same causes, and that in their progress they have, *passibus æquis*, proceeded together, the propriety of these principles will be incontestibly and irremoveably established.

The

The diftinguifhing marks of fcrophula are thus defcribed by Doctor Cullen. *"Glandularum conglobatarum, præfertim in collo, tumores; labium fuperius, et columna nafi, tumida; facies florida; cutis levis; tumidum abdomen."** The defcriptions of Sauvage, Linnæus, and Vogel, are nearly fimilar, but as they are given with much brevity, I fhall here tranfcribe them for the fatisfaction of thofe who may not have obferved them. *" Tumor fchirrofus glandularum colli, mefenteriique, cum labiis, et nafo craffioribus.* Sauvage, G. 21. *Tumor glandularum colli, et mefenterii indolens, obduratus."* Vogel 367. *" Glandula infarcta. Nodus indolens, folidiufculus, preffione obtufe fentiens."* Linnæus 284.

The

---

* Cullen's Synopfis Nofologiæ Method. 79.

The ineſtimable writings of Dr. Cullen afford a very ſtrong teſtimony, that the analogy between ſcrophula and phthiſis, is moſt commonly to be traced. The whole tenor of his chapter on the phthiſis pulmonalis* ſeems to argue, that a ſcrophulous diatheſis accompanies, or rather gives birth to, the diſeaſe. The noxious acrimony which appears in one caſe, and that too a very frequent one, of phthiſis, according to his opinion, is of the ſame kind with that which is obſerved to prevail univerſally in ſcrophula. He obſerves that a phthiſis, at its uſual period, frequently attacks perſons born of ſcrophulous parents; that very often when the phthiſis appears, there occur, at the ſame time,

* Vide Firſt Lines of the Practice of Phyſic, V. 2. C. IV. S. 1.

time, some lymphatic tumors in the external parts. *Glandularum conglobatarum, præsertim in collo, tumores:* and he has also found, very often, the tabes mesenterica joined with the phthisis pulmonalis. He further observes, that, even when no scrophulous affection has either manifestly preceded, or accompanied phthisis, this disease, however, most commonly affects persons of a habit resembling the scrophulous. He describes these to be persons of a sanguine, or sanguineo-melancholic temperament, having fine skins, rosy complexions, large veins, soft flesh, and a thick upper lip; which is almost a literal translation of a considerable part of his definition of scrophula; *Labium superius tumidum: facies florida: cutis levis.* Thus it appears that scrophulous and phthisical persons are originally

originally possessed of the same external conformation of body, and that the dispositions inherent in them are nearly, if not precisely the same. The only dissimilitude which I have been able to ascertain between them, and which by no means can be considered to constitute any essential difference in the characters of these diseases, is in the time of their attack: scrophula being for the most part, observable in the earlier part of life, and phthisis at a more advanced period. In fact, therefore, the phthisis pulmonalis seems to me to be nothing more than scrophula arrived at the years of maturity; more formidable certainly in its advanced age than in its infancy, in proportion as the seat of its affection is of greater importance to life, than the diseased glands of an earlier period; and

cæteris

cæteris paribus more difficult of cure, as it has acquired strength and obstinacy by its duration.

The best histories of scrophula teach us that laxity and delicacy of fibre, are the distinguishing features of persons who are subject to it. The same appearances constantly mark the predisposition to phthisis pulmonalis. The circumscribed redness of the cheeks, and other symptoms of plethora, are equally common to both diseases. This plethora is the immediate consequence of that laxity of the muscular fibres, which, pervading the whole of the vascular system, occasions the blood vessels to admit a larger quantity of blood into them, than, in their natural condition, they are capable of receiving; and

produces

produces that local congeftion in the face, and that diftention of the veins, which are found to accompany fcrophulous and phthifical patients: and this condition is in direct oppofition to the nature of inflammatory diathefis, which confifts of an increafed tone, and contractility of the mufcular fibres of the vafcular fyftem, and produces denfity and conftriction, inftead of laxity and diftention of the affected veffels.

The enlargement of the glandular fyftem, which takes place both in fcrophula, and phthifis, is produced in the fame manner. There is a manifeft atony of the affected parts, which are notoriously indolent, and torpid, and, unlike inflammatory affections, which are accompanied with throbbing pain, heat, and rapid suppuration, are scarcely, if at all painful, and if they suppurate, the progress is remarkably tedious, and requires the aid of the most stimulating treatment to accelerate and promote it.

This is illustrated by observing what happens in any common phlegmon, which, by the by, seldom happens but in persons of a firm and robust constitution. The progress of this, accompanied with tension, heat, and considerable pain, is so rapid, that in spite of all that can be attempted to check it, it will run through all its stages, and form a complete abscess in a very few days. On the contrary, the glandular affections of scrophulous and phthisical habits, if they suppurate at all, (which is not frequently the cafe,) take as many weeks to effect it, and inftead of an antiphlogiftic treatment, a liberal ufe of the bark is requifite, to aid and affift the fuppurative procefs. Inflammation, it is true, accompanies both cafes; but it is widely different in its nature. In the former, the veffels are full of tone, and their action is morbidly increafed: In the latter, there is an evident atony, and laxity of the veffels, and their action is morbidly diminifhed. Hence arifes the different indications of cure in thefe cafes, and it is upon this foundation that the practice is eftablifhed, which I fhall defcribe in the next chapter, and which, hereafter, I fhall attempt more fully to explain.

CHAP.

CHAP. 3d.

TO remove the scrophulous diathesis of the system, to obviate the tendency to atonic inflammation, and to correct a vitious purulency of the affected organ, embraces the whole of the indication of cure upon the principles I have laid down; and as a manifest debility appears to be materially connected with, if it be not the entire cause of, all these symptoms, the following method of treatment, arising out of it, is that which I presume to recommend, and which has been, in the foregoing cases, so successfully adopted.

I have generally premifed an emetic of ipecacuanha, accommodating the dofe to the circumftances of age and condition, and varying the repetition of it as the exigency of the cafe required.

I have fometimes given the folution of Vitriolum Romanum, as recommended by Dr. Simmons, but, upon the whole, I have found reafon to prefer ipecacuanha, which, under all circumftances, is the moft fafe and effectual medicine of the emetic clafs.

The emetic may be repeated, at the diftance of from three days to a week, feveral times, and the following medicines adminiftered during the intervals.

R   *Infuſi*

R *Infusi Corticis Peruviani unciam cum semisse,*
Tinct: Cort: P: Comp: drachmas duas,
—— Lavend: C:
Syr: Cort: Aurantii ana drachmam,
Pulv: Gummi Myrrhæ grana xv, M.
signetur haustus bis quotidie sumendus.

The state of the bowels should be attended to in the mean time with great care; if costive, they should be opened by some gentle laxative, such as tamarinds, chrystals of tartar, or infusion of senna: If on the contrary, a small portion of Gum Arabic, aromatic confection, or an opiate, should be added to the draught. If the cough should be particularly troublesome, the following medicine may be succesfully exhibited.

R *Pil.*

R *Pilulæ e Scilla*

——— *ex Opio ana grana quinque, fiant duæ pilulæ h. f. exhibendæ, et cum dimidia Opii quantitate mane iterandæ.*

To obviate occafional pains of the thorax, blifters ought to be applied, and renewed as often as fhall appear neceffary; and to defend the furface of the body againft the viciffitudes of temperature, and the injuries of cold and moifture, a flannel covering fhould always be recommended.

If the ftrength of the patient be not too far exhaufted, riding on horfeback fhould be ftrictly injoined, which cannot be too frequently ufed. And if the weaknefs fhould be fo confiderable as to render this exercife impracticable,

impracticable, fwinging, in the manner defcribed by Dr. Carmichael Smyth, fhould be fubftituted, and regularly ufed once or twice every day.

If the irritability of the body be very confiderable, the opiate may be given during the day, at convenient intervals, and the dofe gradually increafed, as the habit of ufing it diminifhes its effect. I have feen the *Tinctura Opii* given in dofes of from forty to feventy drops, three times a day, with wonderful good effect.

Should the colliquative difcharge by the fkin prove troublefome, the dofe of myrrh may be increafed; and if it continue obftinate, moderate quantities of the vitriolic acid,

acid, given in some cold draught, will be found a useful remedy. In some of the cases already related, the patient has been taken out of bed, upon the appearance of the sweat taking place, and the *Infusum Rosæ, cum Acido Vitrioli,* administered with great advantage. Cold port wine and water, has also been found very efficacious in checking this inordinate and enervating discharge.

The best time of administering the emetic will be about an hour previous to the evening exacerbation. I have seen the hectic paroxysm prevented by its operation, and the cough and dyspnœa surprisingly relieved. Expectoration is greatly facilitated also by the operation of vomiting, and if care be taken, to prevent the fatigue and relaxation consequent

ON PULMONARY CONSUMPTIONS. 49

confequent upon the exertion it occafions, by adminiftering fome cordial draught immediately after it, vomiting will moft commonly produce confiderable benefit.

In conformity with this general plan, a nutrient regimen is to be adopted. Animal food, that is eafy of digeftion, as it contains more of the principle of nourifhment than vegetable, will be preferable to it. Where the ftomach will bear it, folid meats, of a plain fort, are admiffible; in other cafes, broths and jellies muft be fubftituted. Oyfters, either raw or roafted, and eggs whofe whites are fcarcely coagulated by boiling, have been ufed, in many inftances, with great advantage. Milk has alfo generally made a part of the regimen in the cafes which

G I have

I have attended: and where it has not happened to offend the ſtomach, (which is often the caſe,) it has appeared to afford ſufficient nouriſhment. The addition of rum, or any other ardent ſpirit, I conſider to be uſeleſs, and injurious. Spirituous liquors, of all kinds, have a tendency to increaſe the irritation of coughing, and by deſtroying the tone of the ſtomach, add to the general relaxation of the body, aggravate the hectic paroxyſms, and augment the debility of the ſyſtem. This does not happen with wine, or well fermented malt liquor. Of the former, a glaſs may be taken four or five times during the day; and of the latter, a draught taken occaſionally as common drink. Porter poſſeſſes a generous quality, and diſagrees with but few phthiſical patients. I have generally found

ON PULMONARY CONSUMPTIONS. 51

found it very grateful to the ſtomachs of thoſe to whom I have recommended it, and I have ſeldom ſeen any inconvenience ariſing from its uſe.

I have frequently given the mixture of myrrh and ſteel, ſo highly extolled by the late Dr. Griffith, and have obſerved great benefit to accrue from it. It is, however, ſo extremely unpleaſant, both in color and taſte, that I have ſeldom been able to prevail upon thoſe, for whom I have directed it, to perſevere in its uſe any conſiderable time.

I have ſometimes varied the combination, in order to obviate theſe objections to its uſe, in the following manner.

R *Extract*

R *Extracti Cort: Peruv: grana decem,*
Ferri Vitriolati grana quinque,
Bals: Peruviani q. f. ut fiant pilulæ tres;
horifque medicinalibus, bis de die fumantur, cum
hauftu fequenti.

R *Mifturæ Salinæ uncias duas,*
Pulv: Gummi Myrrhæ grana decem, M.

If the myrrh be mixed while the effervefcence continues, and the draught fwallowed immediately, not only the tafte is rendered much lefs difagreeable, but the efficacy of the medicine is increafed, by conveying along with it into the ftomach, a portion of fixed air, which as an antifeptic, and tonic, poffeffes great virtues, and cannot

not fail to co-operate with the general plan of cure eftablifhed upon this principle.

This medicine was given by Doctor Percival, in the manner thus defcribed, to one of thofe patients, whofe cafes he has related in the memoirs of the London Medical Society, and in fome communication with which he has favored me on the fubject, he has fpoken of it in terms of high commendation.

CHAP. 4th.

I Shall now beg leave to add a very few obfervations on the fubject of the methods

thods above recommended, which will lead, I hope, both to explain the cauſe of ſome inconveniencies which they occaſionally produce, and ſuggeſt the means of removing them.

The bark, in ſubſtance, is apt to occaſion much uneaſineſs in the region of the ſtomach, nauſea, and difficulty of breathing.

In the caſe, related p. 6 of this work, ſoon after the patient had taken the bark, which was adminiſtered in ſubſtance, ſhe diſcovered a ſenſe of weight and pain at the epigaſtrium, accompanied with nauſea. The uſe of the bark was, therefore, ſuſpended, and an emetic exhibited, by the operation of which, a quantity of powder of bark, in a palpable

palpable form, was rejected, made into a firm mafs, with a glutinous matter in the ftomach, the evacuation of which removed the troublefome fymptoms above-mentioned.

This accumulation of the bark, when given in fubftance, has not unfrequently happened under circumftances attending a debilitated condition of the digeftive organs, and has been the caufe of much uneafinefs, and complaint. The difficulty of breathing, and oppreffion which it has occafioned, have been falfely attributed to inflammatory ob- ftructions of the lungs, and other parts of the cheft, in confequence of the operation of the bark. The fact is, that the whole of the inconvenience which the bark, thus ad- miniftered, is apt to occafion, originates in
the

the ſtomach, and, as in other caſes of dyſ-pepſia, is owing to the want of its due digeſtion and aſſimilation; in conſequence of this defect of digeſtion, a fermentative proceſs takes place in the ſtomach, and produces diſtention and oppreſſion of that organ, head-ache, difficulty of breathing, flatulency, and a long train of dyſpeptic ſymptoms. As the pathology of thoſe ſymptoms is evident, ſo is their remedy. Let the ſtomach be evacuated by a gentle emetic, and afterwards, the bark be adminiſtered, either in decoction, or infuſion. I have generally preferred a cold infuſion, prepared with calcareous earth, as deſcribed and recommended by my late valuable friend Dr. Thomas Skeete, Phyſician to Guy's Hoſpital, the Aſylum, and the Finſbury Diſpenſary, in his work on the uſe of

ON PULMONARY CONSUMPTIONS. 57

of the bark, and I have feldom been difappointed in the expectation of its fuccefs. I have, in a variety of cafes, feen as good effects produced by the bark adminiftered in this form, as could have been expected from the fubftance itfelf.

Vomiting, if it be confidered merely as an evacuant, would appear inconfiftent with the principles I have attempted to inculcate as the foundation of a tonic plan of treatment in pulmonary confumptions. The effects of vomiting, however, are by no means confined to the evacuation produced by it, which, in my opinion, conftitutes the moft inconfiderable and unimportant part of its operation. Full vomiting, though it will eventually debilitate, (as every other general agitation

tion of the fyftem will do,) does, by a primary operation, give tone, vigour, and excitement, both to the ftomach, and the fyftem at large: if, therefore, the excitement produced by the primary operation of full vomiting, be in any degree fuftained by a judicious exhibition of fome mild ftimulant and tonic remedies, immediately upon the ceafing of the emetic operation, the efficacy of repeated vomits, in cafes of this kind, and, indeed, in all diforders of great weaknefs, will be fufficiently obvious. In phthifical cafes, efpecially, while they have the general good effects of roufing the energy of the fyftem, and removing the impediments to the digeftion and affimilation of that fubftance which is fo neceffary for the fupport and nourifhment of the exhaufted body, they are alfo calculated

calculated to be of the utmoſt utility as expectorants; and, in my opinion, there is no medicine to which the appellation of expectorant can with ſo much propriety be applied; for by the action of the pectoral and intercoſtal muſcles, together with the compreſſion of the air in the cavity of the lungs by the ſhutting of the glottis, which neceſſarily happens in the effort of vomiting, expectoration is more effectually promoted than by any other means that I am acquainted with.

The uſe of opium, in the caſes related, and in the large doſes in which it has been adminiſtered, will appear to many a practice of great temerity, and to require ſome explanation, or at leaſt, an apology.

With

With respect to the actual mode of its operation, how, in various persons, such various effects are produced, so that in one instance it shall appear to induce immediate and profound sleep, and in another watchfulness, and even delirium, it is not our present business to enquire.

Doctor Huxham, who was, to apply his own nervous language to himself, *Asclepiadeæ Familiæ, dum viveret, egregium Decus et Ornamentum,* speaking of opium, makes the following observation. "*Quod ad opium attinet nihil certi statui potest; cum ipsissima dosis alterum soporet maxime, alteri det contra dulce furere.**

This

---

* *Huxham De Aere et Morbis Epidemicis. Vide de Colicæ Damnoniorum Opusculum.* P. 32.

ON PULMONARY CONSUMPTIONS. 61

This queſtion, which has of late years been ſo much agitated in the ſchools of medicine, ſeems ſtill to remain *ſub judice*. Nothing has ever created more difference of opinion amongſt medical men, than the *modus operandi* of this famous article of the materia medica; and no ſubject has ever ſuffered a ſeverer ſcrutiny; notwithſtanding which, a decided opinion of the preciſe operation of this remedy, or of the diſeaſes to which it is applicable, has not yet been eſtabliſhed. Its great and powerful virtues are, at the ſame time, admitted on all ſides, and that without its aſſiſtance, *manca fit et claudicet medicina*, ſeems to be an univerſal opinion.

From a very reſpectable authority we are informed, " that it induces a dullneſs of the ſenſes,

senses, renders the pulse less frequent, and the respiration slower; that it diminishes animal heat, and checks all the secretions and excretions, except perspiration; that it constipates the belly, and impedes the functions of the stomach; and the same authority instructs us, "*omnes igitur ejus effectus ex vi sedante explicandi veniunt.*"*

From another authority, of great respectability also, we are taught to form a very different conclusion. " That opium acts by a stimulating quality, appears from its effects when given in an over-dose, ‡ or when applied

---

* Vide *De Usu Opii, &c. Diss. Inaug. Auct.* R. B. Remmett. 1773, *edit. Edinburghi.*

‡ *Laudanum Opiatum purgans. Ephem. Nat. Cur. Decad.* 2d. T. 8. P. 117.

applied to a very fore inflamed part. In the firft cafe it produces vomiting and convulfions; in the laft excruciating pain.* Now was its action purely and effentially anodyne, it would be anodyne in all circumftances whatever: the greater its dofe, and the more the nerve was expofed to its action, the more certainly would it fucceed in abating pain. We may venture, therefore, to conclude, that it produces fleep, juft as onions and tobacco do, in confequence of a particular mode and degree of irritation.‡

While there is fuch a wide difference of opinion between men who have beftowed fo much

---

* Schenkius Lib. 1ft. Cap. 296.
‡ Vide Speculations and Conjectures on the Qualities of the Nerves, by S. Mufgrave, M. D. &c.

much labor and ſtudy upon the ſubject, I may be allowed, without the imputation of arrogance, to entertain an opinion which is the reſult of my own experience, and which has taught me to adminiſter opium, in the diſeaſe under our conſideration, without the leaſt apprehenſion of any injurious effects from it.

The cough is ever a moſt harraſſing ſymptom; it deſtroys the reſt of the patient, and wonderfully exhauſts his ſtrength. I adminiſtered opium, therefore, on this account, and I have not yet found any means ſo effectual of allaying this diſtreſſing ſymptom. It has the further good effect of reconciling the ſtomach to the operation of thoſe medicines which I have found to be indiſpenſably neceſſary, neceffary, and which, without its affiftance, could not be fo adminiftered as to produce any permanent good effect. That it checks expectoration, fo as to occafion any material inconvenience, I have never experienced, nor can I believe. The moft troublefome cough, accompanying phthifis, is more frequently produced by the irritation of tubercles, or fome acrid defluxion upon the lungs, than by the extravafation of purulent matter, which, if it be effufed into the bronchiæ, will be expectorated though opium be adminiftered ever fo freely; and it is furely much better that the matter to be expectorated fhould be allowed to collect itfelf in a certain quantity, and evacuated by an effectual cough, twice or thrice in the twenty-four hours, than that the patient fhould be perpetually

harraffed

harraffed with an irritating cough, to throw it up *guttatim*, as it is fecreted, and diftilled into the cavities of the lungs.

If it fhould be further objected to the ufe of opium, that it is calculated to increafe the tendency to the inflammation of tubercles, in the incipient, or more advanced ftages of phthifis pulmonalis, in which I have directed it, I muft refer to the fubfequent part of this work for a defence of the practice; in which I fhall endeavor to prove that fuch an inflammation does not require an antiphlogiftic regimen; that it is an inflammation depending upon an atonic ftate of the fyftem; accompanied, probably, with a fcrophulous diathefis; and that it muft be obviated by an anodyne, and tonic method of treatment,

treatment, of which opium makes a necessary and important part.

The utility of the mode of exercise which I have recommended, has been so entirely confirmed by the experience already quoted, that it would be an unnecessary waste of time to dwell longer upon this part of the treatment. The cases related by Dr. Smyth afford a testimony of its efficacy* beyond the possibility of doubt and uncertainty. They exhibit also a proof incontrovertible, *a posteriori*, both of the atonic character of the disease, and the possibility of its cure, even in its most advanced stages. With respect to the good effects also of riding on horseback,

* Vide Essay on the Effects of Swinging in Consumptions of the Lungs, by J. C. Smyth, M. D. &c.

back, in the incipient state of the disease, the instances I have related are corroborated by indubitable facts, and sanctioned by the opinion of unquestionable authority. In an essay on phthisis, published some years ago by Doctor Simmons,* a case is related of a young man affected with a phthisical cough, and other alarming symptoms, who was effectually cured by a long journey on horseback, from Maidstone to Edinburgh, and from thence to London, which was performed in a very short space of time.

The immortal Sydenham also, speaking of this exercise, makes use of the following nervous, and enthusiastic language.

" *Quantumcunque*

* Vide Essay on Consumptions, &c. by Samuel Foart Simmons, M. D. F. R. S. &c. London.

" Quantumcunque exitialis phthifis et fit et audiat, utpote qua intereunt duo fere trientes eorum quos morbi chronici jugulant, hoc tamen sancte affero, quod neque cortex Peruvianus in intermittentibus, neque mercurius in lue venerea efficaciores extent, quam in phthifi curanda exercitium jam laudatum.*

CHAP. 5th.

THE eftablifhed method of treatment in confumptive complaints is fo generally known that it is unneceffary for me here to give it in detail.

The ufe of an antiphlogiftic regimen, abftinence,

* Vide *Sydenhami Opera*, 8vo. Londini, 1765. P. 383, et 364.

ſtinence, bleeding, demulcent and expectorant medicines, have, for a ſeries of years, conſtituted the principal part of the treatment of phthiſical patients, and this practice has been inculcated by great authority, and confirmed by almoſt univerſal uſage; that it has been frequently ſuccefsful, its warmeſt advocates have not even inſinuated; the contrary is notoriouſly true, and the annals of this miſerable diſeaſe, amidſt a long liſt of caſes too affecting to be recited, afford a hiſtory of recoveries lamentably conciſe indeed. So very unſuccefsful have the ordinary methods of treatment been found, and ſuch has been the fatality generally attending the diſeaſe, that independently of all theoretical diſquiſition concerning it, and ſetting aſide every other conſideration, theſe alone might have

have been thought fufficient reafons for adopting other methods; nor could any practice, under fuch circumftances, be juftly ftigmatized with the imputation of idle experiment, or wanton temerity.

If the colour of any rational principle could have been found to favor a method of treatment differing in fome meafure from that which had hitherto been fo unfuccefsfully practifed, who could have been fufpected of feeling the flighteft objection to whatever deviation it might have fuggefted ? Is it not moft probable, that fuch a deviation would have been adopted with eagernefs, and if that had been found equally ineffectual, that the induftry of mankind would ftill have been exerted to difcover other, and more happy expedients ?

expedients? In such a pursuit, some useful discovery might reasonably have been expected, and even if reiterated trials had still been attended with new disappointment, some benefit might yet have been derived from successive labours. *Felix quem faciunt aliena pericula cautum.*

It is my intention, in this chapter, to endeavor to exhibit not merely the colour of a rational principle upon which a practice materially different from that which has been established is founded, but a real, a substantial, and, I trust, a convincing proof of its propriety. I submit my endeavors to the candid reader for his deliberate judgement; I request that they may be fairly and duly confidered; and I sincerely desire that they

may

may have the effect of exciting in him the ardor of inveſtigation that may lead to the further improvement of a ſyſtem which I conſider ſtill to labor under great and important difficulties. I ſhall reap the fruits of ſuch inveſtigation, in common with my brethren of the faculty, who are intereſted as I am, in the honor of the profeſſion, and who deſire, as I do, to promote, what is intimately connected with it, the general welfare of mankind. Solicitous to be confirmed in the opinions I entertain on this ſubject, if they ſhall be found right, and willing to correct whatever in them may be erroneous, I addreſs myſelf to him in the language of Horace, with the ſincere interpretation of its meaning: *Si quid novisti rectius istis candidus imperti; si non his utere mecum.*

The greatest difficulty that has occurred on the subject of treating the phthisis pulmonalis with tonic remedies, has been the inflammatory affection of the lungs preceding, and accompanying the disease. Of this the occasional hardness, and constant frequency of the pulse, pain of the chest, difficulty of breathing, flushing of the face, &c. have been considered as unquestionable pathognomonic symptoms. If the question respecting the existence of an inflammatory diathesis depended entirely upon these symptoms, I could no longer entertain any doubt of its being the case, as they do, more or less, attend every disease of this kind: but I object

ject to the conclusion, that these symptoms afford any proof whatever of a phlogistic diathesis of the system. On the contrary, frequency of the pulse is invariably a symptom of an atonic state of the body; it occurs, most commonly, in cases of fever depending on debility; in typhous fever, erysipelatous and other exanthematous diseases; while in the synocha, and other affections of a truly phlogistic diathesis, the frequency of the pulse is little, if at all increased. The difficulty of breathing is a symptom still less conclusive with respect to an inflammatory condition of the chest. If the cases of pleuritis and peripneumony be excepted, there is scarcely any pneumonic affection accompanied with this symptom, in which atony and spasm are not evidently to be traced. In

asthma

asthma and dyspnoea this is clearly the case; it also occurs in hypochondriasis, dyspepsia, and an infinite number of instances, recorded by Sauvage and others, in which inflammation has never been suspected. The pain in these cases originates in the same cause as the dyspnoea, and as an individual symptom, affords not the slightest proof of inflammation, but much more frequently indicates a spasmodic affection. *Atonia gignit spasmum* is an adage of Hoffman, the propriety of which is not doubted; that spasm produces pain is a position equally and more generally true.

Of the symptoms then occurring in phthisis, which I have enumerated as the fallacious signs of inflammatory diathesis, the

the occafional hardnefs of the pulfe alone remains to be explained, as it appears that the others are not merely unconfined to inflammatory diforders of the lungs, but are, in fact, much more frequently the offspring of an affection totally different both in its nature and method of cure. This hardnefs of the pulfe, if it were an uniform and perpetual fymptom, would indeed go a great way in eftablifhing the probability of the exiftence of inflammatory diathefis in thefe cafes, and of the confequent neceffity of an antiphlogiftic regimen. But this is by no means the cafe. The hardnefs of the pulfe is not conftant; it occurs at intervals only; previous to fome hæmorrhagy probably, or in confequence of fome other caufe which has operated to excite the reaction of the fyftem,

of

of which alone this can be confidered to be a fymptom. Whatever tends to roufe the reaction of the fyftem, or in other words to excite the action of the *Vis Medicatrix Naturæ*, may occafion fome degree of hardnefs in the pulfe. The common effects of violent exercife, any fudden emotion of mind, or any act of intemperance, is an illuftration of this. The fame happens in epilepfy, and other convulfive, and fpafmodic difeafes. The fame, alfo, occurs in intermittent fevers, in which, though almoft all the characteriftic features of inflammation have contrived to affemble themfelves together, no rational man will be prompted to have recourfe to an antiphlogiftic practice.

Having thus briefly examined the fymptoms

toms which have generally been confidered as the indications of a cooling, or antiphlogiftic mode of treatment, in the difeafe under our confideration, I proceed to enquire how far it is probable, or even poffible, that a ftate of the veffels requiring fuch treatment, can exift in this difeafe. Confiftently with the received opinions with refpect to the pathology of phthifis, and the definition of an inflammatory diathefis, as it is given us by the beft authority, it is both improbable, and impoffible. Dr. Cullen defcribes the phthifis pulmonalis in the following manner; *Corporis emaciatio et debilitas, cum expectoratione purulenta,* accompanied with hectic fever. Of the phlogiftic diathefis he fays, " I define it to be an increafe of tone and contractility of the whole arterial fyftem."*

Can

* Cullen's Firft Lines of the Practice of Phyfic.

Can the tone of the whole arterial fyftem, and the contractility depending upon it, be increafed while the body is in a ftate of emaciation and debility? The arterial fyftem is fo incorporated with every part of the body, that it muft fympathize with it in all circumftances whatfoever. If the body be vigorous, the arterial fyftem will alfo be full of tone and energy. If the body be emaciated and weak, fo muft be the arterial fyftem. Is there then the leaft analogy between the emaciation and debility of the body, accompanying phthifis, and the increafed tone and vigor which conftitute an active inflammatory diathefis?

That there is a fpecies of inflammatory diathefis attending pulmonary confumptions, and

and that the confideration of it is of great importance to the fuccefsful treatment of the difeafe, I am thoroughly perfuaded. The fpecific nature of this inflammation, explains, at once, all the phenomena of phthifis, confirms the theory I prefume to offer on the fubject, and eftablifhes the foundation of the practice I have recommended, upon the folid bafis of a rational principle, as well as fuccefsful experience. This fpecies of inflammation, whether it be fpecifically fcrophulous or not, muft, from the habits of the perfons who are the fubjects of it, as well as the concomitant circumftances of its flow progrefs, and the peculiar organization of the parts it affects, depend upon atony and relaxation of the veffels affected. That there are two kinds of inflammation, and

that

that too, not with flight fhades of difference only, but effentially and diametrically oppofite in their natures to one another, is a fact which I imagine is now univerfally admitted.

That the atonic, paffive, or fcrophulous inflammation is that which accompanies phthifis pulmonalis, is the doctrine for which I contend, and upon which I am folicitous to found a practice whofe nature is fo very different from that which has hitherto obtained almoft univerfal patronage. Nor is there any thing in this doctrine which entitles me to the credit of having made a difcovery, or which has, indeed, any thing of novelty in it, except in its application to this particular form of difeafe. In common fcrophulous

phulous inflammations, originating in laxity, and debility of the affected organs, and of the fyftem at large, whether the mefenteric glands, the large joints, or other parts of the body, have been the feat of the difeafe, practitioners have found no difficulty in recommending the ufe of tonic remedies. We have the beft authority in the records of medicine, with refpect to the efficacy of the Peruvian bark, mezereon, &c. in almoft every form of fcrophulous affections; and as we have feen that the fimilitude between phthifis and fcrophula is fo very ftriking, as to warrant the conclufion, that they are, in fact, no other than varieties of one and the fame difeafe, it muft appear that the indication of cure is neceffarily the fame in either cafe of it.

To

To the want of making a due diſtinction between theſe different kinds of inflammation, has been owing the error in practice which I have attempted to correct, and which appears to me ſo obvious, as to ſtrike, at firſt view, every obſerver. The ſymptoms of pain, heat, redneſs, &c. which are common to all inflammations, have occaſioned the indiſcriminate uſe of an antiphlogiſtic treatment, which has conſiſted chiefly of cooling, and ſedative remedies. How different is this from the practice ſuggeſted by Dr. Percival, who ſays, " that in ſome caſes wine and cordials are the moſt powerful antiphlogiſtics in nature."* He illuſtrates this poſition by an inſtance of the ſucceſsful method of treating the cynanche maligna, and diſorders

* Memoirs of the London Medical Society, V. 2.

ON PULMONARY CONSUMPTIONS. 85

diforders of that clafs, in which this atonic inflammation is very evident; and the doctrine is equally applicable to every fpecies of inflammation, whether general or local, in which debility, and atony appear, as is evidently the cafe in tubercles, and hectic fever, to be the proximate caufe of the difeafe.

When it is confidered that the caufes of inflammation are fo various, and the condition of parts actually labouring under inflammatory affection, are fo widely different as have been ftated above, it will be evident that the indication of cure, under thefe varieties of remote, and proximate caufes, muft alfo materially differ, and that, while bleeding, and an antiphlogiftic regimen, with refrigerant, or debilitating medicines, are neceffary

ceffary in the one cafe, tonic remedies are indifpenfably requifite in the other. To illuftrate this, let us fuppofe a perfon of a found, robuft habit, with a predifpofition to an active inflammatory diathefis, affected with a fimple opthalmia, and let us fuppofe the fame cafe to occur in a perfon of a delicate, or fcrophulous habit of body. The difeafe, in either inftance, is ftill an opthalmia: but is the rational method of treatment alike in both cafes? In the former topical, and perhaps general bleeding, the ufe of lenient purgatives, with cooling and fedative applications to the affected parts, and, in fhort, the whole of the antiphlogiftic regimen will be neceffary. In the latter, not only the local affection will require the aid of tonic, and aftringent applications, but the
additional

additional afliftance of the bark, and every ftrengthening mode of treatment muft be employed in order to effect a cure. Vary this treatment in either of thefe cafes, and the worft confequences will enfue.

The application of this to affections of the lungs is obvious. Efpecially in the cafe under our confideration, it may be urged with much force, and propriety. The habits of phthifical people being, as has been defcribed, extremely delicate, and either actually partaking of a fcrophulous diathefis, or being nearly allied to it, I confider the inflammation which accompanies the fuppuration of tubercles, to be of a fcrophulous nature. Together with this temperament, the nature of the fubftance which is

the

the feat of the inflammation, the flow progrefs of the difeafe, and its concomitant fymptoms of emaciation, and debility, as I have remarked already, all forbid the idea of any active inflammatory diathefis, and are the ftrongeft proofs that can be adduced, amounting, in my opinion, to abfolute confirmation, of the oppofite ftate of the fyftem; of fuch a ftate as requires the ufe of a nourifhing diet, and of cordial and ftrengthening remedies. " *Cibi vero,*" fays Celfus, " *effe debent ex his qui facile concoquuntur, maximeque alunt*; *ergo vini quoque neceffarius ufus.*"*

If thefe premifes be true, what objection can reafonably be made to the ufe of tonic remedies; or rather, what defence can be
fet

* *Celfus de Re Medica.* L. 3. C. 22.

set up of the oppofite practice, whofe object is to diminifh the powers of the body already in a ftate of great debility, under the miftaken idea of removing inflammation, of which that very debility is the caufe? *Sublata caufa tollitur effectus*, is an adage which is as applicable to the practice of medicine, as to any other branch of philofophy. The principal object of a good practice is to afcertain what is the precife nature of the caufe of any morbid affection. This is the great *defideratum* of our art. When that knowledge is obtained, the treatment is obvious, and a material ftep is made towards the cure: without it, whatever practice is adopted muft be uncertain, empirical, and dangerous.

It may frequently happen, however, that when

when the precife nature of the proximate caufe cannot be developed, fome collateral circumftances may afford fufficient hints for the eftablifhment of the curative indication in particular cafes, and for the general guidance of our practice.

In the difeafe under our confideration, I think this is peculiarly the cafe; even admitting that the fcrophulous diathefis of phthifical patients is not univerfally the cafe, and if it were, that the fcrophula itfelf has never yet been accurately and fatisfactorily explained, ftill I think no difficulty would be thrown in the way of the conclufions I have drawn, refpecting the propriety of ufing tonic remedies.

ON PULMONARY CONSUMPTIONS. 91

To afcertain whether an inflammation be of an active, and phlogiftic nature, or whether it be of a paffive, and atonic kind, can never be a matter of any confiderable difficulty. The features of phlogiftic diathefis are very characteriftic, and cannot eafily be miftaken. A firm robuft conftitution, the character of which is fufficiently notorious, is alone fubject to the former defcription of inflammation. Perfons of a weak and delicate fibre are the fubjects of the latter fpecies. This obfervation will be found to apply, very extenfively, to difeafes in general; and I cannot too forcibly recommend the principle of it to the attention of practitioners. Hippocrates has founded fome of his admirable aphorifms upon the fame general principle, and their propriety has never been doubted.

doubted. If I might take the liberty to offer a general obfervation upon this fubject, in imitation of his example, without fubjecting myfelf to the charge of affectation, it would be the following.

Perfons of a weak, delicate, and irritable conftitution, are never fubject to a truly inflammatory diathefis. The inflammation to which fuch conftitutions are liable, is of an atonic or fcrophulous kind, and muft be removed by tonic remedies. On the contrary, the active inflammatory diathefis, confifting of an increafed tone, and contractility of the vafcular fyftem, attacks thofe only who poffefs a firm, and vigorous habit of body, and requires to be treated by what is called the antiphlogiftic regimen; which regimen

principally

principally confifts in the means of leffening the tone of the mufcular fibres, and diminifhing the energy of the fyftem.

CONCLUSION.

HAVING profecuted the confideration of this fubject to a fufficient length, before I entirely difmifs it, I fhall beg leave to fuggeft a few obfervations which may lead to a comparifon between the effects of the method of treatment which has refulted from the doctrine contained in this effay, and thofe of the eftablifhed practice of former times.

In thefe cafes which have come immediately under my own obfervation, and in thofe which I have related from authorities of indifputable veracity, a very refpectable lift of recoveries is exhibited, from fituations of great difficulty and danger, in all of which the method of treatment which I have here recommended has been made ufe of.

In the former annals of this difeafe, from the earlieft periods of medical hiftory, to the prefent times, fuch favorable accounts are very rarely to be met with; fo rarely, indeed, that in all the books I have read on the fubject, (and I have made a diligent fearch into this part of the hiftory of medicine,) I have fcarcely met with one well authenticated cafe of a perfect recovery obtained

ON PULMONARY CONSUMPTIONS. 95

tained by the former mode of treatment. The Edinburgh Medical Eſſays and Communications, the laborious compilations of a very extenſive ſociety, afford one or two inſtances only, and theſe too of an anomalous kind. I have been equally diſappointed in ſearching the miſcellaneous eſſays of later times for information on the ſubject, nor have the combined labours of Morgagni, Bonetus, or Hoffman, afforded me any ſatisfactory proofs of the efficacy of the antiphlogiſtic mode of treatment which has been the faſhion of preceding times.

The late Dr. Dovar has, indeed, affected to relate ſurpriſing inſtances of the good effects of repeated bleeding, in the treatment of pulmonary conſumption; and I ſhould have

have a poor claim upon thofe into whofe hands this effay may fall, for their belief of the facts contained in it, fhould I declare the difficulties I feel in giving entire credit to his moft extraordinary accounts. I fhould be ftill more open to the charge of illiberality, were I to dwell upon thofe cafes, in which a very fpeedy and fatal termination feems to have been produced by the practice which I confider fo very erroneous. Waving the further confideration of this unpleafant part of the fubject, it muft appear evident, that the fuccefsful events of thofe cafes which, during the laft five or fix years, have appeared in the records of our fcience, have far exceeded thofe which former times have exhibited; and as the difference of treatment has already been fufficiently pointed out,

out, I fhall leave the reader to make his own conclufions upon the fubject. If it be fairly inveftigated, that the decifion will be in favor of the fyftem which I have, however imperfectly, attempted to inculcate, I have great reafon to expect; and I repeat my wifh, that this work may operate as an incitement to the further, and more ample inveftigation of the fubject. The neceffity of this is manifeft; for fuch are the prejudices in favor of the eftablifhed practice, and fo obftinate are the objections of the majority of practitioners, to whatever appears to innovate upon the confirmed ufage of their predeceffors, that I muft be vain indeed, to hope for any reformation in their practice, from my feeble efforts. Even amongft my friends, I have the misfortune to obferve fome, whofe infatuated attachment to eftablifhed cuftoms, I am unable to fubdue; and while I obferve the infufficiency of my endeavors to promote a reform in this moft important part of the practice of medicine, amongft thofe who are more immediately within the fcope of my influence, I may reafonably entertain my doubts about their fuccefs amongft thofe who are removed fo much farther out of its reach. While, however, I remain fo fully convinced of the neceffity of eftablifhing a reform in this part of the fcience of medicine, I will ftill perfevere in my humble efforts to accomplifh it, arduous and irkfome as the tafk undoubtedly is. I have received great encouragement, in the progrefs of my endeavors, from the countenance of Dr. Percival, Dr. Kentifh, and other eminent

men,

ON PULMONARY CONSUMPTIONS.

men, whofe experience has been of great fatisfaction to me, and the affiftance of whofe labors has greatly favored the progrefs of my defigns.

While I lament the obftacles to the introduction of what I conceive to be an improved practice in the difeafe which is the fubject of this differtation, amongft the more enlightened part of medical men, I cannot help obferving, that I have found the difficulty to be ftill greater amongft thofe whofe opportunities of gaining information have been lefs extenfive. This indeed is not at all furprifing, when it is confidered that the degree of prejudice, and of pertinacious adherence to a man's own opinion, is generally proportioned to the want of information, and

not

not to the abundance of it, and that the force of a man's obſtinacy is generally to be eſtimated by the weakneſs of his underſtanding.

I met with an inſtance of this not long ago, when I had the unhappineſs to be conſulted in a caſe in which my reputation had nearly ſuffered, together with my feelings. The patient who had been for ſome time gradually ſinking under the preſſure of the moſt violent ſymptoms, which had undoubtedly been greatly aggravated by reiterated bleedings, and the obſervance of a ſlight antiphlogiſtic regimen, died a few days after my viſiting him. The practice of bleeding had been perſevered in till within ten days of this alarming period, while pus had been long expectorated in large quantities, the

patient

patient emaciated to a skeleton, and continually worn out with profuse colliquation. The cordial medicines which I found it necessary to recommend, came too late to do him any service, and the odium of his death was attempted to be thrown upon the ineffectual operation of these medicines, in order to prevent the disgrace that otherwise might have fallen upon the methods which had previously been adopted.

The practice of bleeding has acquired a dangerous reputation in these cases from the temporary relief which it sometimes occasions. This may account in some measure for its prevalence: how the other parts of this description of treatment have obtained so general a patronage, is to be explained in no

other

other way than by the fuppofition of an active inflammatory diathefis having been imagined to give rife to the difeafe; a theory which I hope has been in great meafure, if not entirely, invalidated, by the obfervations which have gone before.

That the practice of bleeding has never been found fuccefsful in a true phthifis pulmonalis, I am firmly perfuaded. That the other

Note. It is to the practice of venæfection too frequently repeated, and in any confiderable quantity, that I particularly object. With refpect to fmall bleedings at diftant intervals, though I have never obferved any permanent good effects produced by them, as they give temporary relief from urgent fymptoms, I think much evil is not to be apprehended, if a tonic and antifpafmodic plan of treatment be allowed to accompany them. The repetition of the operation of bleeding, other parts of an antiphlogiftic regimen have been equally ineffectual in the attempts which have

ing, however, certainly occafions a plethora, and that too of fuch a fort, as feems calculated to excite apprehenfion of its confequences. The manner in which this is produced is defcribed very fatisfactorily by Doctor Cullen, and though his theory on the fubject may appear fomewhat fublimated, it is certainly a rational one, and his conclufions are clear and decifive. The fact feems to have been known, however, before the principle was at all explained, as it has been long the cuftom to bleed cattle occafionally in order to promote their fattening. How it fhould happen that the drawing away this vital fluid, the pabulum of life and energy, fhould difpofe to fatnefs, I will not hazard any attempt to explain. I hope to fee this done by fome who may have experienced the falutary effects of its operation in this way. This operation, however, has feldom, I am afraid, been ufed upon any other principle than that of obviating the fuppofed inflammation indicated by the fizy appearance of the

have been made to cure it by such means, I am equally convinced: and with the idea I entertain

the blood, which is a common, though not an invariable symptom in phthisical patients. How very vague and fallacious this symptom is, when unaccompanied with the other phenomena of inflammatory disease, the experiments of the late ingenious Mr. Hewson will convince any one who will take the trouble to consult them. Among the other phenomena attending the separation of blood after blood letting, it frequently happens that the first or second cup is covered with an inflammatory crust, which is not found in any of the subsequent. Mr. Hewson observed this difference even when there was no difference in the velocity with which the stream issued during the operation, (to which it has commonly been attributed) and when all the other circumstances of the patient were the same as at the commencement of the operation. He is therefore of opinion, that the properties of the blood itself are changed during the operation. If this be the case, the uncertainty, and danger of considering the appearance of the blood as a criterion of any particular morbid

entertain of the nature of the difeafe, which I truſt is founded upon very good grounds, and which certainly has been the refult of extenſive enquiry, and deliberate judgement, I can never believe that fuch methods will be found ferviceable.

On the contrary, while I am perfuaded that a conſiderable degree of weakneſs never fails to accompany the caufes of the difeafe, and

morbid condition of the body are fufficiently obvious. Of other fudden and remarkable changes in the blood, and other fluids of the body, from ſlight caufes affecting the nervous fyſtem, we have fome extraordinary inſtances in the experiments of Baron Haller, and in the obfervations of Hildanus, of which an intereſting account is given in Dr. Mufgrave's admirable book, entitled Conjectures, &c. on the Quality of the Nerves. Vide C. 3. P. 61, and 69.

and that it is very probable that the fame kind of weaknefs, varying perhaps in modification, and degree, conftitutes a material part of the difeafe itfelf, I cannot but confider that fuch means are abfolutely pernicious.

I may be told, perhaps, that inftances have exifted of cures performed by means of bleeding only; or accompanied at leaft by the moft cooling, and debilitating medicines; I can believe it poffible that, under fome circumftances of fpafmodic affection of the cheft, or perhaps fome permanent rheumatic affection, attended with catarrhous fymptoms of confiderable duration, bleeding alone, or fo accompanied, may have effected a cure; but I have never yet feen any thing which could

could induce me to expect that the pulmonary confumption could be cured in this manner; and fuch is my perfuafion of the uniform, and inevitable mortality of this mode of treatment, that fhould a cafe of recovery under fuch circumftances, ever occur to me, I fhould confider it as being next to a miracle, and very ferioufly parody the fentiment of the poet, " time was that when the blood was out a man would die."

Thefe are not the effufions of a warm imagination. I have written from a conviction of the truth of my opinions. The theory I have offered in fupport of them is undoubtedly a rational one. The practice which it points out is confirmed by the unqueftionable authority of fuccefsful experience.

F I N I S.

CONTENTS.

DEDICATION.

INTRODUCTION. ——— *P. i ad xxxii.*

CHAP. I.

Histories of several Cases of Pulmonary Consumption, in which Recoveries were obtained by the tonic Plan of Treatment. ——— 1 *ad* 33

CHAP. II.

A brief Enquiry into the History of Scrophula, with an Attempt to ascertain the Analogy it has with the Habits of phthisical Persons. ——— 33 *ad* 42

CHAP. III.

General Indication of Cure in Phthisis Pulmonalis, with a concise Account of the Remedies used in the above mentioned Cases. ——— 42 *ad* 53

CHAP.

CONTENTS.

CHAP. IV.

Observations on the Effects of some of the Medicines administered, and on the Means of obviating the occasional Inconvenience of their Operation. P. 53 ad 69

CHAP. V.

An Enquiry into the Nature of those Symptoms in Phthisis Pulmonalis assuming the fallacious Appearance of an active Phlogistic Diathesis, with Observations on the Abuse of Blood-letting, and other Parts of the Antiphlogistic Regimen, according to the established Method of treating the Disease ——— ——— ——— 69 ad 93

Conclusion, P. 93, *ad finem.*

www.ingramcontent.com/pod-product-compliance
Lightning Source LLC
Chambersburg PA
CBHW030339170426
43202CB00010B/1174